THE REFLEXOLOGY HANDBOOK

Understanding The Art And Science Of Reflexology: The Reflex Zone Revolution

DEAN OTTO

Contents

Introductory

In reflexology, a kind of complementary medicine, pressure is applied to particular areas on the feet, hands, or ears in order to induce a state of calm and harmony throughout the body. Reflexology is founded on the idea that certain areas of the body, or "zones," correlate to various systems and organs.

The fundamental principle of reflexology is that the body has its own unique channels via which energy flows. A reflexologist's goal in applying pressure to certain spots on the body is to promote harmony and balance by opening energy channels.

Some important things to remember regarding reflexology are:

• Although the feet are the typical targets of reflexology treatments, the hands and ears are not out of the question either. According to popular belief, each section represents a different bodily system.

• Methods: When working with reflex points, reflexologists employ a variety of techniques, such as walking with the thumb or fingers, kneading, and providing pressure.

As a rule, there is a definite and methodical approach to applying the pressure.

- Positive Effects: Those who practice reflexology often report feeling more at peace, less anxious, with better blood flow and general health. Additionally, reflexology can help with some medical conditions and symptoms for some people.

- Holistic Approach: Reflexology takes a more comprehensive approach, treating the full person instead of merely their symptoms. As a complimentary method, it is frequently utilized alongside conventional medical treatment.

• Personal Experiences: Everyone reacts differently to reflexology. Even though some people say they feel better and more relaxed after a session, others could not feel a thing.

While many report feeling better after a reflexology session, there is little proof that the technique actually helps with any particular health issues. While most people feel safe having reflexology done by certified experts, those with specific medical issues should talk to their doctor first.

You should go into reflexology, like any supplementary or alternative medicine, with an open mind and discuss your health issues and objectives with trained professionals.

CHAPTER ONE
Positive Effects Of Reflexology

Many people describe a variety of good outcomes after reflexology treatments, while there is limited scientific data on the precise health advantages. Reflexology is not meant to replace regular medical treatment, and it's important to remember that everyone reacts differently. People often associate reflexology with the following potential benefits:

• Deep relaxation is one of the most frequently mentioned advantages. If you're feeling anxious or stressed out, reflexology may be just what you need to relax and unwind.

- A lot of people find that reflexology helps them deal with stress and worry. Both the mental and physical tolls of stress may be lessened by the treatment's calming effects.

- Many people feel that by applying pressure to specific locations on their bodies, known as reflex points, they can improve circulation. There are a number of systems and organs that may gain from better circulation.

• Some people find that reflexology helps alleviate pain, especially in specific regions of the body like the foot. It may not get to the root of the pain, but it could help with the discomfort and make you feel better overall.

• Improved Sleep: Reflexology is occasionally used to help people have a better night's rest. Those who have trouble sleeping or relaxing at night may find relief from its calming effects.

• Reflexologists frequently talk about restoring harmony to the body's energy systems.

Theoretically, the body's energy pathways can be brought back into harmony by stimulating specific places called reflex points.

• As an additional kind of treatment, reflexology can be helpful for certain people with a variety of medical disorders, including gastrointestinal problems, headaches, and hormone imbalances. Nevertheless, for a holistic approach to health, it is essential to seek advice from a healthcare practitioner.

• Enhanced Well-Being: Reflexology has a way of making individuals feel better all around. It is possible to have a pleasant and relaxing experience by combining physical touch with relaxation techniques and paying close attention to certain parts of the body.

Before beginning reflexology, it is important to establish reasonable expectations and to discuss any health concerns openly with a trained reflexologist.

Many individuals find reflexology relaxing and enjoyable, but whether or not it really helps with certain health problems is something that scientists and doctors are currently debating.

It is recommended that you get advice from a healthcare expert if you have particular health concerns.

The Mechanism Of Reflexology

There is a lack of scientific data demonstrating the effectiveness of reflexology, and the precise process by which it operates is also not fully known. Supporters and practitioners of reflexology, on the other hand, offer a number of hypotheses regarding the modality's potential physiological effects:

• Some people practice reflexology with the belief that certain areas on the feet, hands, and ears are associated with particular bodily systems and organs. The goal of applying pressure to these locations, known as reflex points, is to encourage the flow of energy and provide harmony to the related systems and organs.

• Reflexology is believed to stimulate the peripheral nervous system by the application of pressure on the skin. Some areas of the body may react once this kind of stimulus reaches the central nervous system.

• Endorphin Release: Endorphins are endogenous chemicals that the body produces in response to pain and other positive emotions. They may be stimulated by the pressure applied during reflexology. Many people report feeling more relaxed and less stressed following reflexology sessions, and this may be one reason why.

• Some people think that reflexology can improve circulation and blood flow. The transport of oxygen and nutrients to cells as well as the elimination of waste materials may be aided by better circulation.

• Harmonizing Energy Routes: Meridians, channels, or energy pathways are widely used in holistic health systems, including traditional Chinese medicine, to describe the movement of life force energy. Some people believe that by balancing and opening these energy pathways, reflexology can improve their health and well-being in general.

• Reduced Stress Hormones and Optimal Physiological and Mental Health: Reflexology's sedative effects have the potential to set off the body's relaxation response.

Despite the many reports of beneficial effects from reflexology, there is a dearth of evidence about the exact processes by which it works or if it is effective in addressing specific medical issues. When done by qualified professionals, reflexology is usually safe, but it is not a replacement for regular medical treatment.

Seek the advice of a trained reflexologist and be completely honest about any health issues you may be experiencing if you're thinking about getting reflexology. It is also important to go to a doctor if you have any preexisting health issues to make sure reflexology is a good fit for you as a supplemental therapy.

CHAPTER TWO
Areas & Points For Reflexology

A key tenet of reflexology is the idea that various sites on the body's meridians represent different systems, organs, and structures.

To apply pressure and induce energy flow, reflexologists use these zones and points. Although reflexology is most often performed on the feet, it can also be applied to the hands and ears. A brief outline of the reflexology points and zones is as follows.

1. Ground level:

• It is believed that the spine corresponds to the inside and outside margins of the foot. There is an inner curve that corresponds to the spine, and an outer curve that corresponds to the other edge.

• The great toe is thought to stand in for the brain, while the tips of the toes are said to correlate to the skull.

• The heart and chest region are linked to the ball of the foot.

• It is believed that the digestive organs are associated with the arch of the foot.

• The heel is frequently associated with the pelvis and lower back.

2. The hands:

• Just like the feet, the hands also have reflex points. The head is represented by the tips of the fingers, while the upper torso and chest are symbolized by the palm.

3. Listening area:

• Reflex sites in the ear are believed to represent the complete body. A reflexologist may target certain parts of the ear that are associated with different bodily systems and organs.

Reflexology sessions involve a variety of techniques, such as kneading, pressing, and thumb or finger walking on certain particular spots. In most cases, the pressure is given in a methodical and focused way to help with relaxation, energy flow, and general health.

It's worth noting that different reflexology traditions and practitioners may use slightly different maps and organ associations when it comes to reflexology.

Even though many individuals appreciate reflexology for its calming effects, there is little scientific evidence to back up the specific mapping of points and their effectiveness in treating particular health issues. If you are curious about giving reflexology a try, it is recommended that you find a professional reflexologist.

Standard Reflexology Procedures

Although it has ancient origins, reflexology really came into its own as a supplementary and alternative medicine in the twentieth century, thanks to a number of guiding principles. Reflexology is based on the following principles:

1. Organ and System Correspondences with Reflex Points:

• The practice of reflexology is based on the idea that various sites on the body—including the feet, hands, and ears—correspond to various systems, glands, and organs. "Reflex points" or "zones" describe these specific locations.

2. Unblocking Energy Flow:

- Reflexology is based on the principle that the body has its own unique channels for the movement of life energy, which is also called Qi or prana. It is thought that disruptions or imbalances in the flow of this energy are the root causes of illness or discomfort.

3. Harmony and Energization:

- Reflexology's principal objective is to increase the body's internal energy flow and harmony by stimulating these reflex spots.

Practitioners seek to alleviate stress, open energy channels, and promote a restoration to balance by applying pressure to specific locations on the body known as reflex points.

4. Comprehensive Strategy:

• As a comprehensive therapy, reflexology focuses on the complete individual, not merely their symptoms. The interdependence of the physical, mental, and spiritual realms is considered.

5. Lessening Tension and Relaxation:

• One common way to unwind is with reflexology. It is thought that the pressure used during a session might help people relax and unwind, which in turn reduces tension and stress.

6. Alternative Medicine:

• As a complementary therapy, reflexology often works in tandem with more traditional medical approaches. Instead than taking the place of medical treatment, it should be used to supplement and improve health in general.

7. Tailored Approach:

• The methodology of a reflexologist is customized to meet the specific requirements of each client. The client's symptoms and health issues will determine which reflex sites will be targeted.

8. Anatomy of the Reflex Zone:

- There are certain regions of the body that correlate to each of the reflex zones that traverse the body. Maps of the feet, hands, and ears are utilized by reflexologists to demarcate these zones and locations.

It's worth mentioning that although many individuals like reflexology for its calming effects, there is minimal scientific evidence to back its precise methods and effectiveness in treating certain health issues. When done by qualified specialists, reflexology is usually safe, but for a more thorough approach to one's health, it's best to see a doctor.

CHAPTER THREE
Getting Ready For A Reflexology Treatment

You can make sure you'll have a pleasant and relaxing reflexology session by following these procedures before your appointment. In order to get the most out of your reflexology session, consider the following:

1. Find a Reflexologist Who Meets Your Needs:

• Seek out a reflexologist who is both trained and insured. Before hiring them, make sure you look over their ratings, credentials, and certifications. Get referrals from people you know in the medical field or ask for personal recommendations from people you know.

2. Wear Clothes That Provide Comfort:

• Make sure to wear loose-fitting, comfy garments that provide you easy access to your lower legs and feet. Wearing loose-fitting clothing that allows you to easily reach your hands is a good idea in case your reflexology session includes hand work.

3. Keep Yourself Clean:

• Wash your hands thoroughly before the session to maintain appropriate personal hygiene. Because the reflexologist will be touching your feet directly, it is imperative that they be clean.

4. Please provide your medical history:

• Make sure the reflexologist is aware of any preexisting ailments, drugs, or operations you may have recently undergone. If the reflexologist knows about any sensitive regions on your body, they can adjust the treatment accordingly.

5. Talk About Your Objectives and Worries:

• Discuss your objectives and any particular worries you might have with the reflexologist prior to your appointment. By communicating your goals for the session, such as stress reduction, relaxation, or assistance with a specific health concern, the reflexologist will be able to tailor the treatment to your needs.

6. Ways to De-Stress:

• If you're having trouble unwinding before your session, try practicing relaxation techniques. To enhance your reflexology experience, try deep breathing, meditation, or light stretching to relax your mind.

7. Stay well hydrated:

• Make sure to stay hydrated before the session by drinking plenty of water. In addition to enhancing the treatment's efficacy, staying properly hydrated can aid in the elimination of toxins produced during the session.

8. Eat Moderately:

• Have light snacks and water before your session. One way to ease any pain associated with reflexology is to eat lightly before the therapy.

9. Show Up Early:

• Get to your appointment a little early so you can fill out any paperwork and get settled in. This will make sure that the session may begin promptly and without any unnecessary haste.

10. Unwind While We Are Meeting:

• Concentrate on unwinding once the session starts. Relax and enjoy the reflexology session; just make sure to let the reflexologist know what pressure works best for you.

Reflexology is a complimentary treatment, so keep in mind that although it helps some people, it can work differently for others. Before attempting reflexology or any alternative therapy, it is wise to talk to a doctor if you have any health issues or concerns.

Implements And Gear

When applying pressure to the reflex points, reflexologists usually use their hands, fingers, and thumbs. But, if you want to take your reflexology to the next level or cater to a particular need, you may use the following supplementary instruments and equipment:

1. Lotion or Oil for Massage:

• To eliminate friction and achieve more fluid movements, some reflexologists apply massage oil or lotion. In general, it can make you feel more relaxed.

2. Sink or Tub for the Feet:

• Clients may be requested to soak their feet in warm water prior to a reflexology session. In order to facilitate the reflexology therapy, this can assist loosen up the muscles in the feet.

3. Alternative to cornstarch or talc:

• To make the reflexology treatment go more smoothly, reflexologists sometimes apply cornstarch or talcum powder on the feet to minimize friction.

4. Maps & Charts for Reflexology:

• When diagnosing reflex sites and the organs they belong to, reflexologists frequently consult foot, hand, or ear maps or charts. During the session, the practitioner is assisted by these visual aids.

5. Place to Sit or Lean:

• During a reflexology session, clients usually sit on a comfy chair or one that reclines. It is important that the reflexologist has good access to the feet and that the chair provides sufficient support.

6. Soft Surface:

• For the client's comfort, a towel or blanket could be given. Since relaxing is a crucial component of reflexology, it is essential to keep the client warm.

7. Pillows and cushions:

• Clients can be helped to maintain a comfortable position throughout the session by using pillows or cushions to support their back or neck.

8. Cleansing Cloths or Mop:

• In order to keep their hands and feet clean, reflexologists may use towels or sanitary wipes to clean the feet prior to each session.

9. Clock or Timer:

• To keep sessions on track and give clients the full allotted amount of time for therapy, some reflexologists employ clocks or timers.

10. An optional aromatherapy diffuser:

• Essential oil diffusers are used by some reflexologists to add aromatherapy to their treatments. Some aromas could enhance the calming effect.

Although these tools and technology can be utilized, the main emphasis of reflexology lies in the manual stimulation of reflex sites with the fingers and palms.

The particular methods and resources used can also differ from one practitioner to the next based on personal choice. Before scheduling a reflexology session, it's wise to talk to your therapist about your expectations and any issues you may have.

CHAPTER FOUR
Essential Methods

In order to induce calm and harmony in the body, reflexologists use light pressure to particular areas on the feet, hands, or ears. Some of the most fundamental reflexology procedures are as follows:

1. Unsteady Stepping:

• The reflexologist walks over the reflex spots with their thumbs, applying pressure in a fundamental technique. Consistent and rhythmic pressure, typically felt from the heel to the toe, is required.

2. Skipping Fingers:

• As with thumb walking, finger walking entails pressing the reflex spots with the fingers. It's a more exact method that could be useful for tasks requiring finer details.

3. Revolving Pressure:

• Reflexology involves the practitioner pressing particular reflex spots in a circular or rotating motion with their thumbs or fingers. It is common practice to employ this method when aiming to alleviate stress in a specific region.

4. Reducing One's Body Mass:

• When you knead, you gently squeeze and elevate your foot with your hands. The arch and ball of the foot are two common bigger areas that get this treatment. Kneading is a great way to relieve stress and unwind.

5. Secure and Reliable:

• The reflexologist applies pressure to a specific area by first hooking their fingers onto a reflex point, and then they gently retract their fingers before releasing the pressure. For targeted stimulation of certain areas, it may work.

6. Joints that Rotate:

• The reflexologist might use a light touch to gently twist the fingers' or toes' joints. Increased range of motion and less stress on the joints are two benefits of this method.

7. Press and hold with your finger or thumb:

• The therapist may gently push down on a designated reflex area and maintain that position for a brief period of time. It is believed that this static pressure will facilitate the discharge of stress and the movement of energy.

8. Walking with your fingers or thumbs on your hands:

• It is also possible to do reflexology on the hands. The palm and fingers can be used in a similar way as the thumb when walking.

9. Flexibility Exercises:

• Gentle stretching movements are incorporated into the sessions of some reflexologists. The toes can be gently pulled or the foot can be bent and stretched to achieve this.

10. Spinal Reflexes:

• While applying pressure to the appropriate reflex areas, a reflexologist may delicately rotate the patient's ankle or wrist. Joint mobility can be enhanced with this method.

Reflexology treatments require caution and the client's comfort level to determine the appropriate level of pressure. The end goal is to make the person's experience pleasant and helpful. Before scheduling a reflexology appointment, it's important to discuss your needs and preferences honestly with the practitioner.

Acupressure Points For Particular Areas

By applying pressure to certain points on the body, reflexology can alleviate aches and pains and improve general health. A typical reflexology session may involve massaging the whole foot, hand, or ear, but for more specific results, the therapist can choose to concentrate on certain areas or points. The following are some places that can benefit from reflexology:

1. The Sinuses and Head:

• It's common to find reflex sites on the toes that correspond to the head and sinuses. If you're suffering from a headache or sinus congestion, try massaging your toes gently in a circular manner.

2. Shoulders and Neck:

• Usually, you may find the parts of the foot that correlate to the shoulders and neck up top, close to the base of the toes. As a kind of stress relief, reflexologists may knead or walk their thumbs over this area.

3. The back:

• The bones of the feet form a representation of the spinal column. When treating back pain or promoting spinal health, reflexologists may apply pressure to these locations. All the way around the inside, you can use your thumb or fingers to press down.

4. Abdominal Regions:

• The center of the foot is a common site for reflex sites related to the digestive system. Here you can find techniques that promote digestive health, including thumb walking or kneading.

5. Hormones and the Endocrine System:

• The region surrounding the ankles is frequently treated for issues related to the endocrine system, which includes the pituitary gland, adrenal glands, and thyroid. To promote hormonal harmony, these areas may be gently massaged using circular strokes.

6. Respiration and the Lungs:

• On most people, the ball of the foot is where you'll find the reflex sites for the respiratory system and lungs. Supporting respiratory health and making breathing easier are possible goals of reflexology procedures performed in this area.

7. The heart:

• On the foot, just to the left of the chest area, lies the reflex point for the heart. For the benefit of cardiovascular health, this area may be gently massaged.

8. Irrigation and the Kidneys:

• The renal and urine system reflex points are often found in the middle of the foot. Supporting kidney function can be achieved by techniques like thumb walking or finger pressure.

9. Sexual Organs and the Pelvic Region:

• It is common to find reflex points in the area around the ankle and heel that relate to the pelvic area and reproductive organs. Problems with the reproductive system may respond to reflexology in this region.

10. How to De-Stress and Unwind:

• In order to alleviate tension and promote general relaxation, reflexologists may apply pressure to the whole foot. To achieve overall harmony and health, the standard method is to press on each reflex point.

Rest assured, reflexology is just that—a supplementary therapy—and while it can help with some health issues and promote relaxation, it is in no way meant to replace conventional medical treatment.

It is recommended that you talk to your doctor before attempting reflexology if you have any preexisting medical issues. Also, make sure to let the reflexologist know what you want out of your session and what areas you want to concentrate on.

CHAPTER FIVE
Pediatric Reflexology

Under the supervision of an experienced professional, reflexology can be safely administered to children. Children may benefit from this non-invasive and mild treatment in terms of relaxation and general health. When thinking about reflexology for children, keep in mind the following:

1. Lessening Tension and Relaxation:

• Reflexology has the same calming and stress-relieving effects on children as it does on adults. If you're feeling anxious or stressed out, try applying light pressure to specific reflex areas on your feet or hands.

2. Restorative Nights:

• When it comes to helping children sleep better, reflexology has the support of certain parents and professionals. One possible benefit of reflexology is the improvement in the quality of sleep it induces.

3. Help with Digestive Problems:

• To help children who are having problems with things like constipation or gastrointestinal pain, reflexology techniques that focus on the digestive system might be utilized.

4. Alleviating Pain:

• It is possible to alleviate mild aches and pains in youngsters through the practice of reflexology. Nevertheless, the reflexologist must employ delicate approaches to guarantee the child's comfort during the therapy.

5. Energy Harmony:

• It has the potential to restore harmony to the body's energy pathways. Although there is no concrete evidence to support this claim, many parents report that their children feel better following reflexology treatments.

6. Paying Close Attention:

• As an additional strategy to help kids focus and pay attention, reflexology could be worth looking into. It has been seen by several parents that reflexology sessions help their children concentrate better.

7. Cultivating a Mind-Body Bond:

• Being attuned to one's body and how it reacts is fostered through reflexology. This can be a great approach to help kids become more self-aware and establish a link between their minds and bodies.

While thinking about reflexology for kids:

• Make sure the reflexologist you choose has expertise working with children and the necessary credentials before you hire them. The methods they use should be flexible enough to accommodate the child's developmental stage and degree of comfort.

• Open and honest communication is critical when working with children and reflexologists. The session should be conducted in a way that puts the youngster at ease, and parents or guardians should divulge any pertinent medical details.

• Reflexology treatments for adults tend to be longer, while those for children tend to be shorter. It is common practice to modify sessions based on the child's attention span.

• Get the kid's go-ahead before beginning any session to ensure their comfort and safety. At all times, the youngster ought to feel secure and at ease.

• Involvement of Parents: The presence of parents throughout the session is contingent upon the child's age. For the little one, this can mean feeling safe.

Remember that reflexology can't take the place of a doctor's visit. It is recommended that parents seek the advice of a healthcare professional before introducing their child to reflexology or other complementary therapy for specific health concerns.

Using Reflexology While Carrying A Child

It is crucial for pregnant women to exercise caution and seek the advice of a trained reflexologist before attempting reflexology, while the supplementary therapy has the potential to be safe and helpful. When it comes to pregnancy-related aches and pains, many women find that reflexology helps them relax and feel better. When considering reflexology during pregnancy, keep in mind the following:

Factors to Think About:

1. Priority on Safety:

• Before beginning any alternative therapy while pregnant, it is important to contact with your healthcare professional. It is vital to make sure there are no contraindications before having reflexology while pregnant, even though it is typically safe.

2. Professional in Their Field:

• Look for a reflexologist who has worked with expectant mothers before. For the sake of their pregnant clients' safety and comfort, they should know which reflex spots are off-limits and how to modify their techniques accordingly.

3. When it occurs:

• In most cases, reflexology can be safely performed at any point in a pregnant woman's journey. Still, if you want to keep your miscarriage risk to a minimum, you should probably hold off until after the first trimester.

4. Expressing ideas:

• It's important to be honest with your reflexologist regarding your pregnancy, any pains you're feeling, and your general health. Based on your specific requirements, the reflexologist might modify the treatment plan.

5. Layout for Maximum Comfort:

• The pregnant woman can sit comfortably or lie on her side while receiving reflexology. For maximum ease and support, choose a posture that suits you.

Importantly, reflexology should not be used in place of conventional medical treatment. It is important to check with your doctor to be sure reflexology is safe for you to use while pregnant. To make sure the experience is safe and effective, pick a qualified reflexologist who has done pregnant reflexology before.

Elderly People's Reflexology

For the elderly, reflexology may be a soothing and helpful supplementary treatment option. It's a gentle method of relieving stress and promoting health by pressing on certain areas of the body, such as the feet, hands, or ears.

Some things to think about and possible advantages of reflexology for the elderly are as follows:

Factors to Think About:

1. Current Health Situation:

• The patient's current health condition should be taken into account prior to beginning reflexology or other alternative treatment. To make sure reflexology is safe and appropriate for elderly people, who typically have many health issues, it's recommended that they talk to their doctor.

2. Drug Interactions:

• To avoid potential problems, reflexologists should be notified of any drugs that the elderly person is taking. The reflexologist can adjust their procedures to prevent pressing on any places that could be affected by medicines.

3. Convenience and Freedom:

• People who have trouble moving around might modify reflexology to help them. The reflexologist can modify the session to suit the needs of the older person if they have trouble sitting or lying down.

4. Expressing ideas:

• Having an open line of contact between the reflexologist and the older person is vital. Please let the reflexologist know if you have any particular health concerns, pain regions, or session preferences.

5. Methods that are easy:

• Because of the possible fragility of bones and joints, as well as the sensitivity of aging skin, reflexologists who work with the elderly typically employ softer approaches.

Possible Advantages:

1. Enhanced Blood Flow:

• Some people think that reflexology can improve blood flow. By enhancing tissue oxygenation and bolstering general cardiovascular health, improved circulation may be beneficial for the aged.

2. Alleviating Pain:

• Pain in the joints and other aches and pains caused by arthritis are among the many conditions that reflexology has the potential to alleviate. To relax and unwind, try applying light pressure to certain reflex sites.

3. Relief from Stress:

• Reflexology's sedative effects can help lower stress levels, which is especially helpful for the elderly coping with the effects of becoming older.

4. Better Rest:

• A better night's sleep could be one benefit of reflexology. Changes in sleep patterns are common among the elderly, but reflexology offers a non-pharmacological way to help people get a better night's rest.

5. Feeling Better Overall:

• A better mood and general feeling of well-being could be enhanced by reflexology's calming effects and pleasant sensory experience.

6. Pain Relief for Long-Term Illnesses:

• Some long-term health problems, including diabetes, neuropathy, or gastrointestinal problems, may find relief with reflexology, which is especially useful for the elderly.

7.   Enhancement of Self-Awareness:

• Being attuned to one's body and how it reacts is fostered through reflexology. This might be a great approach for seniors to stay in touch with their bodies and practice self-care.

Remember that reflexology can't fix a broken ankle or other significant health problem; see a doctor if you need emergency medical attention. If you are thinking of getting reflexology for an older loved one, be sure to find a trained professional who has expertise treating this population.

The reflexologist's skills should include flexibility, patience, and awareness of the specific challenges that come with getting older.

CHAPTER SIX
Easy Methods For Conducting
Your Own Self-Reflexology

To practice self-reflexology, one places pressure on particular reflex points on one's own body, such as the feet, hands, or ears.

Even though it won't be the same as getting a professional reflexology treatment, it's still a great way to unwind and feel better. A few simple ways to practice self-reflexology are as follows.

Reflexology of the Hands

1. Unsteady Stepping:

• Find a comfortable seat and hold onto something with both hands. A thumb walk over the palm of your hand creates a circular motion. Be careful to apply light pressure all over the surface.

2. Skipping Fingers:

• Drawing parallels to thumb walking, walk in small circles over the palm with your fingers. The palm's center and the tips of the fingers are two of the many places you should direct your attention.

3. Joint Rotation in the Fingers:

• Carefully move your fingers in both directions by rotating them at the joints. Releasing tension and increasing flexibility are two benefits of this.

4. Release the Wrist:

• With the other hand, hold your wrist and gently press down in circular motions with your thumb. Loosen up by circling the wrist.

Auricular Reflexology:

1. Rotating the Toes:

• Take a comfortable seat and elevate one foot. Start by turning your toes in one direction at the joints, and then switch directions. Flexibility can be enhanced in this way.

2. Stepping on the Sole with the Thumb:

• Make tiny, circular movements with your thumb as you walk along the bottom of your foot. Focus on various parts, like the arch, heel, and ball of the foot.

3. The Roll of the Ball:

• Roll out a tennis ball or other small ball and set it on the floor. Gently press down on the ball with the ball of your foot as you roll it. The result can be like a massage.

4. Arch Press:

• Press down on the arch's center point on the foot's sole with your thumb. Hold the pressure for a few seconds before releasing it. If necessary, repeat.

Assessing the Ears:

1. The Earlobe Massage:

• Use your thumb and forefinger to gently rub your earlobes. It is believed that this region is in close proximity to the brain and skull.

2. Extending the Thumb Past the Ear Canal:

• Move your thumb in tiny, circular motions around the outside of your ear. Various points along the edge warrant your attention.

3. Ear Pluck:

• With one hand, grasp the ear's tip, and with the other, grasp the lobe. Using light pressure, gently tug and release the earlobe as you work your way around the ear.

4. Tactile Application to Reflex Areas:

• Locate any areas of the ear that may be tender or sensitive. Press and hold these points with your fingers for a few seconds. Hold and release as needed.

Basic Advice:

• Unwind: Find a comfortable position and focus on deep breathing exercises.

• Regular self-reflexology sessions may have cumulative benefits, so it's important to be consistent. Think about adding it to your weekly or daily schedule.

• Joining in with Your Body: Notice how your body reacts. Pay extra attention to any area that feels especially sensitive or tender.

Always seek the advice of medical experts before attempting any new self-care routine, including self-reflexology. You should consult a medical professional before attempting self-reflexology or any alternative therapy if you are pregnant or have any pre-existing conditions.

Summary

Finally, reflexology is a non-invasive, holistic treatment that can help you relax, balance your energy, and feel better all over by applying pressure to certain points on your feet, hands, or ears. Despite its long history, reflexology only really took off in the 20th century as an alternative medicine practice.

An important tenet of the practice is the idea that different parts of the body are represented by specific reflex points on the feet and hands. The goal of applying pressure to these areas is to promote relaxation, increase energy flow, and establish internal harmony.

Many people find that reflexology helps them relax, reduces stress, and alleviates specific health concerns. Children, pregnant women, the elderly, and people with particular medical needs can all benefit from its adaptability.

It is critical to choose a competent and experienced practitioner when contemplating reflexology. The reflexologist will usually ask the client about their medical history and any concerns they may have during the consultation portion of the session.

After that, the therapist will target particular reflex points using methods like thumb walking, kneading, and finger pressure.

Although many people enjoy reflexology, there is little scientific evidence to back up any particular health claims.

Although most people feel safe having trained practitioners do reflexology on them, those with preexisting health issues should definitely talk to their doctors before attempting the treatment.

For a more comprehensive approach to health, consider combining reflexology with other therapies like massage, aromatherapy, or acupuncture. Ongoing self-care can also be achieved through the practice of self-reflexology techniques in the comfort of one's own home.

Adding reflexology to your wellness routine can help you relax, reduce stress, and feel better overall. Although results may vary from person to person, reflexology is most effective when used in conjunction with other preventative health measures.

Seek the advice of healthcare providers and reflexologists for personalized recommendations based on individual health needs and situations, and always communicate openly with them.

THE END